C000155332

28 days to E

the pain cycle

By Dr Sue Peacock

ISBN: 978-0995459977

Published by Ann Jaloba Publishing,

the moral right of Sue Peacock to be identified as the author has been asserted in accordance with the copyright design and patents act 1988

Note to Readers

The information, including opinion and analysis contained herein are based on the author's personal experiences. The information provided herein should not be used for diagnosing or treating a health problem or disease. Readers are advised to consult a doctor for medical advice. The author and the publisher make no warranties, either expressed or implied, concerning the accuracy, applicability, activeness, reliability or suitability of the contents. If you wish to apply or follow the advice or recommendations mentioned herein, you take full responsibility for your actions. The author and the publisher of this book shall in no event be held liable for any direct, indirect, incidental or other consequential damages arising directly or indirectly from any use of the information contained in this book. All content is for information only and is not warranted for content accuracy or any other implied or explicit purpose.

WHY KEEP A JOURNAL

Keeping a journal is a positive thing! Your journal will help you see how far you have come and be a record of the successes you have achieved. This will help you build on your success further.

Also it's useful to note what hasn't worked for you, so you can learn from all of your experiences; I frequently say to my patients, there is no such thing as failure, only feedback! Sometimes we learn more from our mistakes than we do our successes, so we often need to develop a plan B or C to enable us to move forward.

Journals are great because they highlight things that you CAN do, and things that haven't gone to plan, so you can adapt and deal with them more positively in the future.

This journal aims to provide space to write down your progress, thoughts and feelings. Additionally it offers self-management tips to help you manage your pain, improve your sleep, managing anxiety and depression and provides a few positive affirmations to help you on your way to manage your pain and the effects of your pain effectively.

Wishing you a less pain day

Dr Sue Peacock

HOW TO USE THIS DIARY: PACING AND PLANNING

This diary is designed to help you lessen your pain within One month, 28 days. It sets out a different activity and tip for each day.

You will get the most our of the diary if you set some time aside every day to work through each day's suggestion. Make sure you fill in the journal part. Not only is writing your feelings and plans a good way of psychologically 'fixing' the good helpful things in your life, it is also a good way of tracking what is going on. I hope one of the things you will get out of working through this diary for a month is a picture of your own ups and downs and what works for you. It is about you taking control and working out what is good for you.

Before you start, I want to say a bit about pacing. It is important that, you take things at your own pace, the one which is right for you.

Often when you are in pain, you keep pushing on . . . this is a common mistake, and you may end up in a good day, bad day cycle.

On good days, you may do too much which then increases pain, tiredness or weakness which leads to resting for a few days. During these 'rest days' you may become frustrated and irritable. Then you may feel better again and play 'catch up' which leads you to overdo things again and become trapped in this vicious cycle.

DIFFERENT WAYS TO BREAK THE CYCLE

Pacing by minutes
Think of an activity and how long you can do it before you feel tired, weak or in pain. Cut this length of time in half and gradually build this time up by 30 seconds to one minute until you can go past the original time.

For example, if you can walk for 10 minutes before you feel tired, weak or in pain, cut this back to 5 minutes when you next go for a walk. See how you feel. If all is okay, increase your walk to 6 minutes for the week. If that is okay, try 7 minutes the week after. If it's not okay at 7 minutes, go back to walking for 6 minutes for the week; then increase to 6½ minutes and continue from there.

Pacing by number
You can also pace by number. For example if you have 12 plants to plant in your garden, plant 6. Then, do something completely different. Later, or the next day, plant a few more.

Pacing by grading
A more complex way, is to list all the activities that you do throughout the day right from getting up to going to bed. Go through the list and grade each activity 0=no pain, tiredness – 10= worse pain, tiredness I could imagine. Plan your day so you say, do an activity that is an 8, followed by anything less than 5. Plan rest breaks into your day. We should aim to maintain an even level of activity over the day.

Here are some tips to help:
It is important to keep active as too much resting leads to loss of conduction resulting in stiffer joints and weaker muscles. We should aim to maintain an even level of activity over the day.

1. Change posture / position regularly (sit, walk, stand)

2. Break tasks into smaller chunks. Stop before the pain increases, see previous page.

3. Take frequent short breaks. Spread your activities over the day/over the week.

4. Be prepared to ask for help / delegate jobs / say No.

5. Gradually increase the amount you do as your body gets more tolerant of activity.

Week One Monday

You are the expert in yourself. What works for you?

Learn to self manage. Many people see their health care professionals for treatment, help and support. However, it has been estimated that you may spend on average, less than 3 hours a year with your health professionals, so of the other 8,733 hours you are on your own! There are many tools to help you and we are going to be detailing them in this diary. But often the best ideas come from you. You know yourself best so write YOUR best coping technique on the page opposite.

Your Monday

My best coping technique . . .

Best thing today

What I would change

Remember for next time

Week One Tuesday

There is at least one thing you need to STOP

Accept you have pain. This is not giving up but changing the way you see your role in managing pain. You have to be in control of it, you have to be willing to use self management techniques and do things differently to the way you have managed in the past. Yesterday you thought about your best coping techniques. Today think about what you need to change. Is there a technique you use which does NOT help? It may be something you have been doing for years, but now it is time to ditch it.

Your Tuesday

The coping technique I should drop

Best thing today

What I would change

Remember for next time

Week One Wednesday

If you have to do things which hurt at least split them

Plan your day. Make a list on what you would like to achieve that day. Remember to be flexible and perhaps think about how activities affect your pain levels and try to avoid doing activities together that potentially increase your pain. Plan short breaks throughout the day and take them!

Your Wednesday

The two activities I should avoid doing next to each other are . . .

Best thing today

What I would change

Remember for next time

Week One Thursday

Unfit muscles feel more pain, so get moving

Stretching and Exercise – many people in pain fear this will cause more problems. However, in reality, stretching and exercise decreases pain, as weak and unfit muscles feel more pain than those you are using regularly. Remember start slowly and build up gradually. Speak to your physiotherapist or GP about taking part in exercise.

Your Thursday

The exercise I will do is . . .

Best thing today

What I would change

Remember for next time

Week One Friday

Relax muscles and mind and the pain will lessen

Relaxation is a useful skill to reduce tension in the body and unwinding your mind. Often when we are in pain, we hold our posture differently as the muscles try to protect the painful part of us; which causes us more pain. However the way we hold ourselves becomes like a bad habit and we don't notice we are doing it. There are a whole range of relaxation skills from progressive muscular relaxation to visualisation. You can find more details on our website http://www.apaininthemind.co.uk/

Your Friday

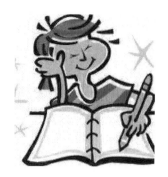

The relaxation technique I will use . .
.

Best thing today

What I would change

Remember for next time

Week One Saturday

Set yourself a goal: swimming in small steps, an example

Set yourself goals. Here is an example using the activity of swimming. If you don't like swimming, apply the ideas to another physical activity which suits you, such as running or walking. Focus on setting realistic goals and break them down in to small chunks. Here is an example which you might even want to start over this weekend. If your goal was to be able to swim 10 lengths of your local pool in 3 months time. This goal could be broken down as follows.

Get a timetable for the swimming pool. Does it have disability sessions where the pool is a little warmer for those sessions?

Decide on a time of day to go, and how many times a week are you going to swim.

Your Saturday

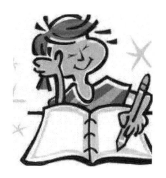

I will decide on my swimming timetable

Best thing today

What I would change

Remember for next time

Week One Sunday

Set yourself a goal: swimming in small steps (2)

Again, if you don't like swimming then you can apply this to another activity. Have you got a friend who will come with you – this sometimes makes it easier to go when your motivation is low.

Have you got a swimming costume, do you still need to buy one?

Visit the pool, check out changing facilities etc.

Go to pool and get in, start to float or just enjoy being in the water.

Swim a width

Swim two widths

Swim a length

Perhaps swim a length and a width

Swim 2 lengths and build up until you have reached your goal of 10 lengths

Celebrate your achievement!

Your Sunday

I will choose a pool and find out details

Best thing today

What I would change

Remember for next time

END OF YOUR WEEK

So take some time and turn the page to reflect on how you have done and plan for next week.

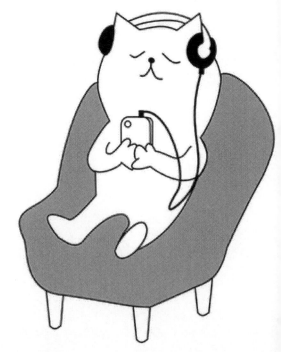

HOW WAS YOUR WEEK?

This is the time to reflect on how it is going, what is

working for you and what you need to adapt

WELCOME THE NEW WEEK

Preparation is all. So note down any challenges or difficult times you know are coming up and have a think about how you will deal with them.

Make sure you have something to look forward to. Write that down here.

AND

Take a look at our website for more resources.

www.apaininthemind.co.uk

Reducing Pain

Week Two Monday

Information is power. Find out everything

If you have been diagnosed with a condition, or have a certain problem which causes you pain, FIND OUT EVERYTHING.

Once you have thought about it, write down all the questions you can think of, discuss them with family/friends and get their inputs. Discuss with your Consultant, GP or other health professional. If you can, take a trusted friend or family member with you to your appointment. Even if these things were discussed at your diagnosis, chances are, you didn't hear them.

Your Monday

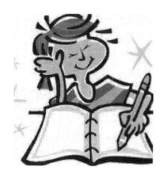

I will find out more about the condition causing my pain

Best thing today

What I would change

Remember for next time

Week Two Tuesday

The breath of life, learn to do it properly

We all breathe all the time, obviously. You may not know that some ways of breathing can help lessen your pain.

Try this one

TRIANGLE BREATHING – draw a triangle, on outer left side, write I, outer right side write E, centre line, write P. I=inhale, E=exhale, P=pause. Use this tool daily. Take a deep breathe in and then blow out. INHALE slowly whilst saying, inhale silently. EXHALE slowly whilst saying, exhale silently. PAUSE 1,2,3,4, then start again.

Your Tuesday

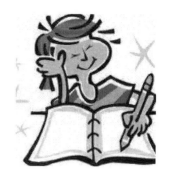

I will draw my breathing triangle and decide what time of day I will use it every day.

Best thing today

What I would change

Remember for next time

Week Two Wednesday

Catch those anxious thoughts before they grow

CATCHING ANXIOUS THOUGHTS – these are thoughts which we continually think about and grow like a snowball. The trick is to catch them before they get bigger. Write down your thoughts, one at a time, see if you can identify ONE thought which started the chain reaction which made you feel so anxious. Keep identifying & writing your thoughts down. Now start with the initial thought and write down a new thought that doesn't result in you feeling anxious. What new thought could you substitute for the first anxious thought? These new thoughts are confident and empowering. Continue working through your lists of thoughts.

Your Wednesday

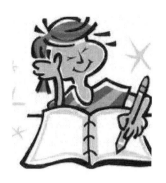

I will make a thoughts list and identify and change at least ONE thought

Best thing today

What I would change

Remember for next time

Week Two Thursday

Visualise yourself away from your pain

I bet you can think of a time when you were so engaged you forgot about your pain. You can use this natural ability to train yourself in distraction techniques. These can be anything from breathing exercises all the way through to hypnosis.

Here is one example, visualisation is a good distraction. However it needs practise before you need it. For example if your are experiencing an increase in pain, think about your favourite place, think about absolutely everything about it, colours, smells, textures, noises etc., practise so you have a really good recall of this place.

Your Thursday

I will decide on my special visualisation and practise it

Best thing today

What I would change

Remember for next time

Week Two Friday

Use what you know calms you to calm you anytime

Stress and anxiety make pain feel worse. If you learn to use those things which you know calm you, then you can help control that pain.

So learn BRINGING CALM BACK. Ask yourself, what would feel really good right now? Then do it.

- A cup of tea?

- Another pillow?

- Listening to some music?

- Doing some colouring?

Your Friday

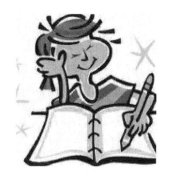

I will write a list of things which calm me for use whenever I need it

Best thing today

What I would change

Remember for next time

Week Two Saturday

Controlling anxious thoughts: stay grounded

Whenever you experience high anxiety KEEP YOURSELF GROUNDED.

To do this use the world around you to stop those anxious thoughts in their tracks.

Look around you, what can you see right now, what colour is the floor, the walls, how many tables are there, what are the light fittings like, are they dusty? What's the person like next to you? Being very focused on another set of thoughts interrupts a chain of anxious thoughts.

Your Saturday

I will practise concentrating on my immediate surroundings

Best thing today

What I would change

Remember for next time

Week Two Sunday

Controlling anxious thoughts (2): the five minutes trick

I CAN'T HANDLE THIS - yes you can! You can handle what's going on for the next 5 minutes, you can do anything for 5 minutes at a time.

Start by using the grounding technique from yesterday. Then catch your anxious thoughts (Wednesday) and visualise a relaxing (and distracting) scene. (Thursday). Finally, use your favourite Bringing Back Calm thing (Friday).

There, 5 minutes have gone

Your Sunday

I will congratulate myself on how much control I am taking

Best thing today

What I would change

Remember for next time

END OF YOUR WEEK

So take some time and turn the page to reflect on how you have done and plan for next week.

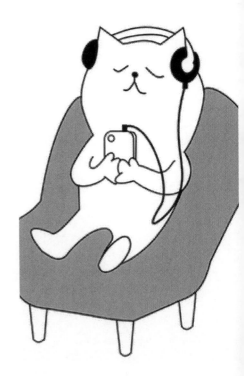

HOW WAS YOUR WEEK?

This is the time to reflect on how it is going, what is

working for you and what you need to adapt

WELCOME THE NEW WEEK

Preparation is all. So note down any challenges or difficult times you know are coming up and have a think about how you will deal with them.

Make sure you have something to look forward to. Write that down here.

AND

Take a look at our website where you will find more information and resources.

www.apaininthemind.co.uk

Reducing Pain

Week Three Monday

Get changes in perspective and deal with 'what-ifs'

Whether it is a change in your medical care or a different feeling when you wake up, ups and downs can be scary. Expect many emotional ups and downs and you will deal with them better. Put your focus on the right now, keep in the present, tell yourself "right now, I am . . ." Don't pile on the potential pressure of *what if* thinking.

Your Monday

I will use my distraction techniques to move away from 'what if' thinking

Best thing today

What I would change

Remember for next time

Week Three Tuesday

Routine gives you a sense of control so value it

TRY TO KEEP ROUTINE - get up/go to bed at the same time each day, try to eat your meals at the same time, watch/listen your favourite programme. It's important to do these small things to give you a sense of control when you feel you don't have any.

Your Tuesday

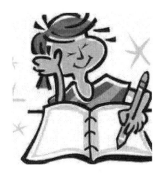

I will write down my routine and try to stick to it

Best thing today

What I would change

Remember for next time

Week Three Wednesday

Concentrate on relationships not pain

RELATIONSHIPS are vital for emotional wellness. Pain can ignite emotions in both your and your loved ones and spill over from one relationship to another. Often pain takes centre stage and that's all you talk about. It is OK to take a break from talking about pain.

Your Wednesday

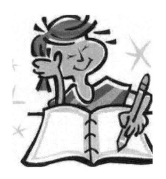

I will set aside a definite time to nurture relationships with my loved ones

Best thing today

What I would change

Remember for next time

Week Three Thursday

You are never alone with a journal, so share your thoughts

THE WORLD GOES ON - while you do have people around you who do care about you, their lives do go on and often this is difficult because you are focused on your pain. This can lead to a deep sense of aloneness, that's normal! Talk about it, journal it, allow yourself to feel what you feel. Writing your feelings down is a way of sharing them.

Your Thursday

I will write down how I am feeling

Best thing today

What I would change

Remember for next time

Week Three Friday

Saying it well: Affirmations can lift your mood

POSITIVE AFFIRMATIONS - write down affirmations you find encouraging, inspiring or helpful, maybe a quote from a famous person or a bible verse, part of a poem or something you have written yourself. A variety of positive affirmations will be helpful depending upon what you are going through at the time.

Your Friday

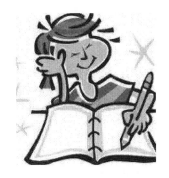

I will collect together my favourite affirmations

Best thing today

What I would change

Remember for next time

Week Three Saturday

The numbers game: making change one at a time

Sometimes change can feel too hard, too big. So take small steps.

MOVE YOURSELF FORWARD ONE NUMBER AT A TIME.

Think of a scale from 1-10, 1=not depressed at all, 10=very depressed. If you are feeling down, give your feeling a number. Then see if you can decrease the number by taking action, turn it into a game, I wonder if I could change it from a 5 to 4?

Your Saturday

I will do one thing to get my 'down feeling' reduced by one number

Best thing today

What I would change

Remember for next time

Week Three Sunday

Take time out from feeling down and you won't feel down

Dealing with your pain can sometimes feel like a full-time job. You are allowed a holiday! So try TIMING OUT. Set a timer for at least 30 mins to give yourself time out. You must use this time to do something pleasurable for you.

Your Sunday

I will take time out and get back in contact with pleasure

Best thing today

What I would change

Remember for next time

END OF YOUR WEEK

So take some time and turn the page to reflect on how you have done and plan for next week.

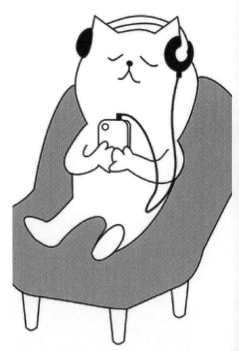

HOW WAS YOUR WEEK?

This is the time to reflect on how it is going, what is

working for you and what you need to adapt

WELCOME THE NEW WEEK

Preparation is all. So note down any challenges or difficult times you know are coming up and have a think about how you will deal with them.

Make sure you have something to look forward to. Write that down here.

Reducing Pain

Week Four Monday

Plan your pleasures: anticipation is a great mood lifter

3 THINGS YOU CAN DO RIGHT NOW - write a list of 3 things you really enjoy doing. Modify them if needs be.

Some examples:

If you want to be outside but can't, move a chair near the window, watch the birds, look at flowers, look at the clouds and make pictures, look at a nature book, watch nature programmes etc. If you can't focus to read, try audiobooks, flick through a magazine, read a short story or poem rather than a long novel. Make a plan of what you enjoy and do that activity, tell your family that's what you are going to do and most importantly DO IT! A key element of taking control is taking action.

Your Monday

I will do 3 things I really enjoy

Best thing today

What I would change

Remember for next time

Week Four Tuesday

Live in the moment and do something good right now

ASK YOURSELF: WHAT CAN I DO FOR MYSELF RIGHT NOW? Call a friend, listen to some music, go out into the garden, take the dog for a walk. This tool often gets ignored when you are caught up in a cycle of pain. If you take action, it can provide surprising and beneficial results.

Your Tuesday

I will be spontaneous and DO SOMETHING

Best thing today

What I would change

Remember for next time

Week Four Wednesday

Be your own best friend and talk to yourself

ENCOURAGING YOURSELF WITH SELF TALK - be compassionate with yourself, acknowledge that it is difficult, but it's ok to feel what you feel, talk to yourself in a kind and supportive way.

Say out loud how you feel when you are on your own. Also say what is good about your life.

Your
Wednesday

I will find a quiet place where I can be alone and talk to myself

Best thing today

What I would change

Remember for next time

Week Four Thursday

The one good goal everyday rule: get good in your life

A 'ME' GOAL EVERY DAY - each day decide on one goal you will achieve for yourself, it can be as simple as reading the paper, checking an email, de-heading a few roses in the garden. Each day write down your goals and write a new one for tomorrow. Looking back at the evidence of achievement & success helps those positive feelings.

Your Thursday

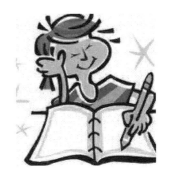

I will decide on some goals which suit me

Best thing today

What I would change

Remember for next time

Week Four Friday

A happy thought is worth remembering: what is yours?

You have a huge store of happiness inside your own head. Your memories.

HAPPY THOUGHT- What one happy thought can you think about? Write it down and bring it to mind throughout the day.

Your Friday

I will write down my 'happy thought' and recall it throughout the day

Best thing today

What I would change

Remember for next time

Week Four Saturday

Stuck is painful, unglue yourself with answers

WHAT'S KEEPING ME STUCK? Sometimes you feel that you can't move on, so write down: what do I think is keeping me stuck?

Do I want more information? If so, what kind of information?

Do I want to make a decision? If so, what decision?

Do I want help with some part? If so, what kind of help, who can help?

Do I need to take action? What action?

Identifying that you are stuck and problem solving how you can move forward is very beneficial.

Your Saturday

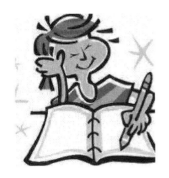

I will make a list of what I need to unstick myself

Best thing today

What I would change

Remember for next time

Week Four Sunday

Your mind, your thoughts and your control

ERASE YOUR 'WHAT IF' THOUGHTS?' - refuse to play the 'what if' game! What if the pain makes me moody and irritable? What if I can't look after myself? One 'what if' thought soon spirals into anxiety. Awareness is the way to stop, ask yourself THESE 2 QUESTIONS:

1. Is this thought helping me or hurting me?

2. Is this thought moving me forward or holding me back?

Your Sunday

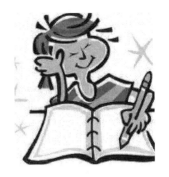

I will keep a list of all my 'what if' thoughts and use everything I have learned to keep them in control

Best thing today

What I would change

Remember for next time

Before you go . . .

Flare-up plans: what to do when things go wrong

At this stage things may be going well and you will be feeling positive about managing your pain. However, we also need to think about the future.

Everyone will continue to have good and bad days or phases. This is unlikely to stop happening altogether.

What *you do* will make a difference to:

- How **often** you have a bad phase or flare-up
- How **long** it lasts
- How **severe** it is at the time

Reducing Pain

Think of your body as a castle
PREVENT A BAD PHASE if possible, by keeping a watch on your (body) castle:

- Prioritise, plan and pace your activity
- Manage your stress i.e., relax
- Exercise and keep active

Flare-ups will happen sometimes and this flare-up plan may help you manage the bad times more effectively.

Plan
1. Recognise early warning signs of trouble on the horizon and take early action
2. Don't panic
3. Recognise and accept that you are in flare-up
4. Bring out your 3 big guns PHYSICAL, PSYCHOLOGICAL, MEDICAL
5. Make managing your flare-up your first and only goal until you feel better

Physical
- Reduce all activities that cause pain
- Exercise very gently if this helps
- Take extra care with posture and standing
- Use warmth/ice/TENS machines if these help
- Wear comfortable clothes that are easy to put on
- After 2-3 days, start to slowly become more active

Medical
- ○ Take your medications as planned and prescribed
- ○ If you are taking tablets make sure you are taking a regular dosage during a bad episode. Don't hang in there until the pain is too much to bear
- ○ Remember that it's a positive skill to use medication correctly and it's a skill that you have learnt

Psychological
- ○ Have confidence in yourself – you know the right things to do to get through this flare-up (if you are experiencing new or different symptoms then check with your GP as well)
- ○ Keep positive. This may be the most difficult part but if you use positive thinking to challenge negative thoughts it will help you to get through the flare-up. "I've got back from this before" . . . "I know it will ease if I use the coping strategies I have learned". . .
- ○ Increase relaxation. Set aside more time to practise relaxation
- ○ Communicate with others. Explain you are in a flare-up and tell them what you are doing to enable you to get back to normal as soon as possible

If you want more help, visit my website

I am at

www.apaininthemind.co.uk

Here you will find

E guides

Audios

Special programmes . . . And much more

Or you can book a session with me

 I will assess your difficulties with you by creating a working partnership – you bring your expertise about you and I will bring my expertise, experience and training in a variety of psychological approaches. Together we will develop a bespoke pain management plan for you.

Contact me at my website and we can start working together.

Goodbye for now and I wish you a pain-free future

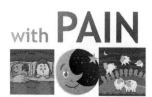

SLEEPING

with PAIN

Strategies for a restful night from pain-management expert

Dr Sue Peacock

Foreword by Pete Moore

PLUS

If you have trouble sleeping, I have written a book especially for you.

Sleeping with Pain: Strategies for a restful night will help you develop habits and strategies to get a good night's rest even if you are in pain.

Readers of *Sleeping with Pain* say:

"This is a wonderful book to take you gradually through steps to help yourself."

"At last a clear straightforward guide to sleep...with pain."

"A really great book, clear and easy to read. Some great thoughts and ideas."

Go to my website to get the book

www.apaininthemind.co.uk

With my best wishes

Dr Sue Peacock

Reducing Pain

Reducing Pain

Printed in Great Britain
by Amazon